DISCOVERING LIFE'S SECRETS
THROUGH FITNESS

WHAT THE FIT

KAPIL MEHROTRA

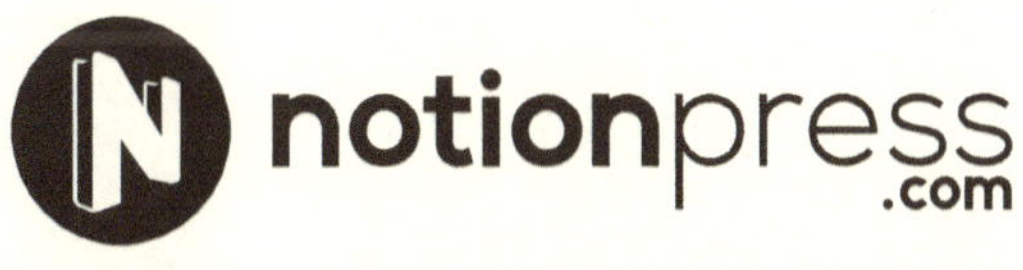

notionpress
.com

INDIA · SINGAPORE · MALAYSIA

Copyright © Kapil Mehrotra 2023
All Rights Reserved.

ISBN 979-8-89067-964-2

This book has been published with all efforts taken to make the material error-free after the consent of the author. However, the author and the publisher do not assume and hereby disclaim any liability to any party for any loss, damage, or disruption caused by errors or omissions, whether such errors or omissions result from negligence, accident, or any other cause.

While every effort has been made to avoid any mistake or omission, this publication is being sold on the condition and understanding that neither the author nor the publishers or printers would be liable in any manner to any person by reason of any mistake or omission in this publication or for any action taken or omitted to be taken or advice rendered or accepted on the basis of this work. For any defect in printing or binding the publishers will be liable only to replace the defective copy by another copy of this work then available.

Contents

Don't trust everything you hear from others. There are always three side to a story: Yours, theirs, and the truth....

– By Kapil Mehrotra

Preface

The pursuit of fitness is an age-old endeavour that transcends borders, cultures, and ideologies. It's a universal aspiration that speaks to our inherent need to feel strong, vital, and empowered. Fitness is more than a regimen; it's a philosophy of life.

This book is more than a guide; it's a transformative journey that invites readers to reimagine their lives from a perspective where fitness is not a mere goal but a way of being. In a world where the corporate grind often leaves individuals feeling disconnected from their bodies and minds, this book offers a pathway to rediscover a sense of wholeness, vitality, and joy.

At its core, the book acknowledges the multidimensional nature of fitness, viewing it not just as a physical endeavour but as a holistic pursuit that integrates mind, body, and spirit. It recognizes the unique challenges and stressors of the urban lifestyle and offers practical, real-world strategies to incorporate wellness into the fabric of everyday life.

It's about finding balance in a world that constantly demands more and learning to align personal and professional life in a way that nourishes the entire self. It's a call to authenticity, resilience, and self-awareness, providing the tools and insights to navigate a complex world with grace, wisdom, and strength.

Whether you are beginning your fitness journey or looking to deepen your understanding of wellness in all its facets, this book is a compass that points the way to a more fulfilling and vibrant life.

Fitness is not a game for showing off, it's a game to compete with yourself...

– By Kapil Mehrotra

Acknowledgements

Embarking on a journey to create a fitness empire is a monumental undertaking, filled with excitement, challenges, collaboration, and determination. The story of Ozone Gym is not merely a tale of brick and mortar, machines and weights, but a narrative that weaves people, passion, culture, and community into a fabric that embodies the essence of fitness.

At this juncture, I must dedicate this book to my incredible and daughter Agrika. Her unwavering support and her own passion for fitness became the spark that ignited my own journey 13 years ago. An astounding individual, a fantastic cook, and a self-made interior designer with not one but two post-graduate degrees, she is a paragon of what one can achieve with dedication. Balancing family life and our two wonderful children,she is the unsung hero behind every word you read, every lesson I've shared

The inception of Ozone Gym was a collaborative endeavor born from friendship and a shared vision. When Mr. Kamal Bagga and Mrs. Ritu Bagga decided to start this elite members club, they were driven not just by a business idea, but by a desire to create a space that fosters well-being, excellence, and camaraderie.

Their vision was to provide superb facilities that went beyond the standard gym experience. They wanted to create an environment that resonated with people's passion for fitness and offered group classes that infused energy and fun into workouts. From Zumba to Bhangra, the intention was to make fitness not just a routine but a celebration.

When I was asked to contribute by setting up group classes and exercise sessions like Zumba and Bhangra, I was thrilled to be a part of this new journey. The gym kicked off well, and people's demands for more classes grew rapidly. My daily visits to the gym became an essential part of my life, transforming from a mere routine into a heartfelt passion.

Kamal Bhaiya's warm welcome each day played a crucial role in fostering my love for the gym, encouraging consistency and commitment. The language of fitness acted as a fast connector, enabling me to meet many amazing elite friends in the gym, who soon became an integral part of my life.

At Ozone, the mission goes beyond mere physical exercise; it's about embracing fitness as a lifestyle. From tailored, personalized training programs to regular, engaging group classes, every aspect of Ozone is thoughtfully designed to cater to the individual needs and goals of each member. Whether a novice looking to take the first steps on their fitness journey or an experienced athlete aiming to push their limits, Ozone is committed to guiding and supporting everyone towards achieving their health and fitness aspirations.

Among the friends and influences from the gym, I'd like to acknowledge Sir Ram Gopal Agarwal Ji, My Boss Rahul Dhanuka Ji, Mrs Ritu Bagga, Mr Kamal Bagga, Ashish Ahuja Bhaiya, Dharam Ahuja Bhaiya, Late Rolly Ahuja Bhabhi, Raghav Arora Bhaiya, Bro Raghav Khanna, Ms Neha Ahuja, Sister Shruti Vaswani, Bro Sajal Seth, Bro

Abhishek Bhateja, Mr India Vinay Kumar Sir, Amit Sir, Rapper Nitin Khatri Sir, Janit Sir, Rohan Sir, Akshay Sir, Running buddy Mahesh R and the entire supporting staff of the gym. Their presence, support, and inspiration were pivotal to my fitness journey, and without them, I could not have achieved what I have. This book draws inspiration from them all, and it is a testament to the incredible impact of the relationships formed at Ozone Gym

Chapter - 1

Stepping Off the Treadmill: Your Transition from Corporate to Fitness

As dawn breaks, the morning sun paints the city in hues of gold, casting long shadows on the deserted streets. The world is still asleep, yet you stand alone, ready to face another day in a world you know all too well - the corporate world. It's a world that thrives on relentless deadlines, unending meetings, and a ceaseless hustle that leaves little room for respite. The humdrum of this existence reverberates in your ears, a monotonous rhythm that has defined your life for far too long.

On this particular morning, however, something is different. As you lace up your shoes and the cool morning air fills your lungs, a stirring of change sweeps over you. In the hush of the dawn, a decision begins to crystallize, hardening with every second that ticks by. It's a decision to embrace change, to shatter the shackles of corporate life, and to embark on a path less trodden. This isn't just another day. It's the start of your revolution, a testament to the indomitable human spirit's ability to reinvent, transform, and ultimately, to thrive.

This book is an intimate exploration of that revolution. It's a journey from the sterile cubicles of corporate offices to the vibrant energy of the gym. It's about breaking barriers, challenging norms, and discovering a new paradigm of health and fitness. It's about finding balance amidst chaos, and harmony amidst discord. It's about your transformation from a corporate employee to a fitness influencer.

Identifying Personal and Professional Challenges

As the first leg in this journey, you confront the realities of your personal and professional life. Both realms are filled with challenges that test your mettle, pushing you to the limits, and eventually, towards change.

Personal Challenges

At home, your roles carry immense weight. As a spouse, you are more than just a partner; you are a cornerstone of support. As a parent, your role extends beyond caregiving to embodying the ideals you wish your children to emulate. As a friend, you are a confidante, a shoulder to lean on during challenging times. Each role demands your time, energy, and emotional bandwidth. The pressure to excel in each and the fear of falling short often create a sense of being overwhelmed.

Professional Challenges

Parallel to this, your professional world presents its unique set of trials. You find yourself in an environment that is as demanding as it is competitive. The hours are gruelling, the workload is relentless, and the deadlines, are unforgiving. Bosses who don't appreciate your efforts and colleagues who don't empathize with your struggles add to the challenges. The constant need to prove your worth fuels your stress, creating an atmosphere that is as difficult to navigate as it is stifling.

However, each of these challenges serves a purpose. They ignite the spark within you for change. They trigger the realization that there's another path, a path towards a healthier, more balanced life. In the chapters that follow, you'll traverse through this transformation, exploring how these challenges metamorphose into opportunities for growth and self-improvement.

The Corporate Quagmire: Understanding Stress Triggers

To navigate away from the corporate world and towards a healthier lifestyle, it is crucial to understand the triggers that contribute to your stress.

Endless Deadlines and Expectations

Your professional world is a maze of deadlines that seem to multiply the closer you get to them. With each project, the expectations grow, not just from your superiors, but also from yourself. The constant race against time creates a relentless cycle of stress that often spills over into your personal life.

Work-Life Imbalance

The boundary between your work and personal life becomes increasingly blurred. You find yourself replying to emails at dinner, thinking about work during family time, and often sacrificing your personal commitments for professional ones. This imbalance, over time, takes a toll on your mental and physical health.

Office Politics and Power Dynamics

I had a boss—someone of stature and formality. He was always impeccably dressed, yet there was a hint of envy in his eyes when he saw how fit I looked in my shirt, tie, and trousers. This jealousy didn't stay hidden; it transformed into a relentless pursuit to keep me chained to my desk well beyond normal working hours.

His attempts to derail my fitness regimen were not merely confined to loading me up with work. He himself embarked on diets, and exercise regimes, and enlisted the support of some female staff, all in a futile attempt to emulate my physique. His endeavours were almost comical, often caught in integrity issues, yet somehow surviving each scandal.

Then there was another boss, a man so driven by his commitments to the MD & CEO that he'd lose all sense of reason and proportion. His crazed desire to meet impossible timelines led to demands that we remain in the office for days on end until the work was completed. His overzealousness knew no bounds, and we often found ourselves caught in his wild toss of unrealistic expectations.

One day, his overreach led to a dramatic unravelling. He was caught red-handed, accepting cuts from IT vendors, his eyes wide with shock and face pale with the realization that his games were up. That moment, etched in memory, was a stark reminder of the absurdities and contradictions that sometimes characterize the corporate world.

The professional world is not just about the work you do but also about the relationships you build and navigate. Office politics, power dynamics, and the constant pressure to conform to the corporate culture add another layer of stress.

The Pursuit of Perfection

In the corporate world, there is often an unspoken expectation to be perfect. Any mistake or failure is seen as a reflection of your capabilities. This pursuit of perfection fosters a fear of failure, making each task a high-stakes game that adds to your stress levels.

Recognizing these stress triggers is a crucial part of your journey. It allows you to understand the factors that impact your well-being and identify the changes you need to make. This understanding forms the foundation of your decision to step away from the corporate world and move towards a lifestyle centred around fitness and wellness. The chapters that follow will explore how you navigated this transformation, turning these stress triggers into motivation for change. Your revolution is gaining momentum.

Envisioning a New Path: The Fitness World

As you delve deeper into the realities of your corporate life, you begin to envision an alternate path. A path that leads away from the stress and strain of the corporate world and towards an environment that fosters health, well-being, and personal growth - the fitness world.

Discovering the Fitness Landscape

Amidst the corporate chaos, you stumble upon a sanctuary - the gym. The gym becomes more than just a place to exercise; it transforms into a haven where you can de-stress, refocus, and rejuvenate. You start exploring different fitness regimes - weight lifting, running, Zumba, yoga - each one opening a new avenue for self-improvement.

Finding Balance through Fitness

You soon discover that fitness is more than just physical well-being; it's a balance of mental, emotional, and spiritual health. The discipline of regular workouts, the mindfulness of yoga, the thrill of running - each activity adds a new facet to your life, helping you find balance amidst the chaos.

Inspiring Change in Others

As your fitness journey progresses, you begin to inspire those around you. You become a beacon of change, encouraging others to embark on their own fitness journeys. The gym transitions from being your sanctuary to a community of like-minded individuals striving for a healthier lifestyle.

"Obstacles may come your way, but don't push them aside. Embrace them, overcome them, and sculpt your strength."

– Kapil Mehrotra

Chapter - 2

Fitness in The Urban Jungle

As the sun peeks through the skyscrapers and the aroma of masala chai wafts through the air, the urban jungle awakens. The rhythmic cacophony of honking cars and the murmurs of busy streets paint the backdrop of a day in the life of an Indian city. Amidst the hustle and bustle, finding moments of serenity can be akin to finding an oasis in a desert. It is here, in this modern concrete labyrinth, that your pursuit of fitness must thrive.

Ah, the mighty local trains of Mumbai! They are akin to the pulsating heartbeat of the city. The symphony of metallic clanks, the roar of engines, and the cacophony of countless voices merge into a melody that is distinctly Mumbai. Here, time waits for no one. The clock ticks as crowds surge through the trains like waves. This is where students, office-goers, dreamers, and fighters, all come together.

Move a little to the east, and Kolkata greets you with the languid charm of yesteryears and the vivacity of today. The buses here are brimming with life and stories. The sweet strains of Rabindra Sangeet may embrace you as you navigate the crowd with your deft movements, something that has become second nature.

Bengaluru, the Silicon Valley of India, is a different challenge altogether. Its vibrant cosmopolitan culture is somewhat overshadowed by the serpentine traffic that seems like a ceaseless river of vehicles. Waiting behind the wheel, the city's salubrious weather keeps you company.

The daily commute is not just a physical journey; it's a mental and emotional marathon. The constant negotiations with auto-wallahs, the endless waiting for buses, and sometimes the sheer proximity to a sea of humanity can be overwhelming.

Yet, within this seemingly mundane routine lies an untapped reservoir of opportunities. When perceived through the lens of creativity and resilience, every minute spent in your daily commute can be a stepping stone towards your fitness goals.

- **The Walks and The Waits:**

  Consider the simple act of walking to the bus stop or the railway station. Can you extend that walk by a few hundred meters? Perhaps alight one stop early and embrace the road on foot. During the endless waits at traffic signals or platforms, can you engage your core, practice deep breathing, or even perform inconspicuous calf raises?

- **The Posture and The Poise:**

  Within the cramped confines of a rickshaw or behind the steering wheel, your posture often takes a beating. Can you consciously rectify that? Draw your shoulders back, straighten your back, and take deep breaths. This not only improves posture but also helps in reducing stress.

- **The Mind and The Music:**

  Commute time can also be a treasure trove for mental wellness. How about indulging in audiobooks or learning a new language through apps? Or even losing yourself in the mystical tunes of Indian classical music or any music that soothes your soul.

- **Mindfulness Practices:**

  Engage in mindfulness practices. While on the bus or train, instead of scrolling endlessly on your phone, try closing your eyes and focusing on your breath, or engage in a short meditation using an app.

- **Positive Affirmations:**

  Amidst the cacophony of honking vehicles and bustling crowds, remind yourself of your strengths and aspirations. Silent positive affirmations can reinforce mental fortitude.

Incorporating Smart Commuting:

While the commute can be used to infuse elements of fitness into your daily life, optimizing and planning your commute smartly can open up opportunities for more structured workouts. Time is the most precious commodity in today's fast-paced world, and saving even a little of it can have a tremendous impact on your lifestyle and fitness.

- **Optimizing Routes and Modes of Transport:**

  Navigating through the urban jungle requires wit and strategy. Consider using route-optimizing apps to find the quickest way to your destination. Sometimes, a combination of transport modes - a bit of walking, followed by a bus ride, and finally a short autorickshaw trip - can save you valuable minutes. Many Indian cities now have Metro services; opting for these can help in avoiding traffic and saving time.

- **Flexible Timings and Carpooling:**

  If your workplace allows, negotiate flexible timings to avoid peak traffic hours. Carpooling is another option to consider. It is not only environmentally friendly but also a fantastic way to build a sense of community. Share your journeys with colleagues, and who knows, you might find a fitness buddy!

- **Remote Working Days:**

  With the advent of technology, the concept of remote working is becoming more prevalent. If possible, work remotely for a few days in a week. The time saved from commuting can be invested in a morning jog, a yoga session, or any fitness activity that you have been longing to try.

Utilize This Saved Time for Workouts

The balancing act of work, family, and personal time is a daunting challenge for many. But what if the secret to incorporating fitness into your life lies not in drastic changes, but in simple, subtle shifts in your daily routine? The Indian ethos is deeply rooted in finding balance and harmony, and it's time to channel this wisdom into your fitness journey.

- **Walking Meetings:**

  Instead of sitting in a conference room, suggest a walking meeting. The gentle exercise is not only good for your health but also for your creativity and problem-solving skills. The rustic charm of Indian streets could very well be the spark that ignites new ideas.

- **Taking the Stairs:**

  Forego the lift and embrace the stairs. Whether at work or at the local shopping centre, choosing stairs is a small change with big benefits. The ancient Indian architectural marvels didn't have elevators, and our ancestors were fitter for them.

- **Homemade Healthy Snacks:**

  Opt for homemade snacks like poha, dhokla, or roasted chana over-packaged products. Traditional Indian snacks are not just flavorful but also packed with nutrients. Carry these to work or have them ready when you get back home.

- **Mindful Eating:**

  Practice mindful eating by savouring each bite, eating slowly, and paying attention to when you are full. Indian cuisine is diverse and rich – make it an experience. Mindful eating can aid in weight management and improve digestion.

- **Active Commute:**

  If possible, cycle or walk to work at least once a week. For longer distances, consider getting off public transport a stop early and walking the rest of the way. This small change can have substantial benefits for your cardiovascular health.

- **Family Activities:**

  Engage in physical activities with your family. Play cricket with your kids or take a family walk after dinner. Not only does this incorporate fitness, but it also strengthens the bonds that are such an integral part of Indian culture.

- **Pause and Breathe:**

  Take short breaks throughout the day to practice deep breathing or meditation. This can help in reducing stress and improving focus. Draw inspiration from the ancient Indian practices of pranayama and meditation.

  Integrating these effortless adjustments into your everyday routine can serve as potent agents for transformation. They embody the diversity and opulence of Indian culture, demonstrating that fitness transcends mere individual pursuit, but rather harmonizes with a well-rounded existence.

"Don't watch the clock; do what it does. Keep going."

– Sam Levenson

Chapter - 3

Shattering Misconceptions: The Reality of Holistic Wellness

As you navigate the urban jungle, turning everyday routines into avenues for fitness, a profound realization sets in. Fitness and wellness encompass more than just physical strength and endurance; they transcend the boundaries of the physical self. They embrace every facet of your existence, from the intellectual to the emotional.

Holistic wellness is an approach to health and well-being that considers the whole person and how they interact with their environment. It's not just about treating specific symptoms or focusing on particular areas of the body. Instead, it considers the whole body and the role it plays in overall health.

The concept of holistic wellness is rooted in the understanding that all aspects of a person's life are interconnected. It acknowledges that physical health, mental well-being and emotional balance.

Physical Wellness: Exercise and Nutrition

Physical wellness is perhaps the most widely recognized aspect of holistic health. It's about taking care of your body to ensure it functions optimally, allowing you to engage fully in life. It encompasses regular physical activity and a nutritious diet, among other practices.

Regular physical activity has a multitude of benefits, from maintaining a healthy weight and reducing the risk of chronic diseases to boosting mood and improving sleep. It's about finding an activity that you enjoy, whether that's yoga, running, weightlifting, dancing, or simply taking a walk in the park. It's about consistency and ensuring that movement becomes a regular part of your lifestyle, not a chore or a tick on a checklist.

Nutrition plays a pivotal role in physical wellness too. The foods you consume can fuel your body, keep your immune system strong, and support your overall health. A balanced diet that includes a variety of nutrients is essential. This means focusing on whole foods - fruits, vegetables, lean proteins, whole grains, and healthy fats - and minimizing processed foods high in sugar, salt, and unhealthy fats. Hydration is another key aspect of nutrition that should not be overlooked.

Keep in mind that it's not about rigidly adhering to a specific diet or following the latest fitness fad. The real focus should be on developing sustainable habits that nurture your long-term health and well-being.

Emotional Wellness: Managing Stress and Fostering Positivity

Emotional wellness goes beyond managing stress and anxiety. It involves recognizing and expressing our feelings, maintaining a positive attitude, and developing resilience in the face of adversity. It's about creating a healthy relationship with our emotions and fostering a positive mindset.

Stress is a normal part of life, but chronic stress can take a toll on our health. It's crucial to develop strategies to manage stress effectively. This might involve mindfulness practices like meditation or yoga, hobbies that help you relax and unwind, or therapy to address deeper emotional issues.

Fostering positivity, meanwhile, doesn't mean ignoring negative emotions or pretending everything is perfect. Rather, it's about recognizing that while we can't control everything that happens to us, we can control how we respond. It's about reframing our perspective, practising gratitude, and developing a growth mindset. It's about focusing on the things that bring us joy and satisfaction and cultivating positivity in our everyday lives.

Emotional wellness is a journey, not a destination. It's about the small steps you take every day to better understand yourself, nurture your mental health, and build a life that aligns with your values and aspirations. It's about being kind to yourself, embracing your emotions, and realizing that it's okay to seek help when you need it.

Debunking Common Misconceptions and Myths

However, the path towards holistic wellness is often shrouded in myths and misconceptions. These misconceptions act as stumbling blocks, clouding your understanding and diluting the essence of wellness. They create illusions of wellness, packaging it into narrow definitions of gym memberships, rigorous workouts, or trending diets. These limited perceptions might lead to temporary gains, but they seldom result in lasting meaningful change.

#1 Eating Healthy Means Starving Yourself

A widely held myth is that eating healthy equates to severely restricting your diet or, worse, starving yourself. This belief, often fueled by unrealistic body standards and diet culture, can lead to unhealthy eating habits and even eating disorders.

The reality is that healthy eating is not about deprivation but about nourishment. It's about providing your body with the nutrients it needs to function optimally, which includes carbohydrates, proteins, fats, vitamins, and minerals.

A healthy diet is balanced and diverse, including a range of foods from different food groups. It does not advocate for the complete exclusion of any food group, including fats and carbs, which often get a bad reputation. In reality, our body needs these for energy and various physiological functions.

Eating healthy also involves listening to your body's signals. It means eating when you're hungry and stopping when you're full. It's not about counting every single calorie but about making more nutritious choices overall.

Importantly, healthy eating is not a one-size-fits-all concept. Each person's body has different nutritional requirements based on age, gender, physical activity level, and overall health. Thus, what works for one person might not necessarily work for another.

So, healthy eating should not be seen as a short-term diet or an unbearable sacrifice but as a long-term lifestyle change that promotes overall health and well-being.

#2 More Gym Time Equals More Fitness

In the realm of fitness myths, the idea that spending more hours in the gym equates to higher levels of fitness is a persistent one. We often see people pushing themselves to exhaustion, believing that longer workouts will lead to quicker or more substantial results. However, this belief is not only misleading but can be counterproductive and even harmful.

First, it's important to understand that the quality of your workout matters more than the quantity. Engaging in a focused, well-rounded exercise routine for a shorter period can be far more beneficial than aimlessly spending hours at the gym.

Second, excessive workouts can lead to overtraining, which can harm your health and fitness goals. Overtraining can cause various issues such as decreased immunity, disturbed sleep, decreased strength and performance, injuries, and even hormonal imbalances.

Third, rest and recovery are as important as exercise in a fitness regimen. Your muscles need time to repair and grow after a workout. Without proper rest, you not only risk injury but also might hamper your progress towards your fitness goals.

Holistic wellness advocates for a balanced lifestyle. Spending disproportionate amounts of time at the gym can disturb this balance, leaving less time for other important aspects of life, such as social activities, hobbies, relaxation, and sleep.

#3 Only High-Intensity Workouts Are Effective

Another common myth is that only high-intensity workouts are effective for improving fitness and losing weight. High-intensity interval training

(HIIT) has gained significant popularity in recent years, leading many to believe that it's the only worthwhile form of exercise.

While HIIT is a highly effective workout method that offers numerous benefits, it's not the only pathway to fitness. Lower-intensity workouts such as brisk walking, swimming, or cycling also offer several health benefits. These activities can improve cardiovascular health, boost mood, assist in weight management, and increase overall stamina and strength.

Moreover, high-intensity workouts may not be suitable for everyone. They can increase the risk of injury, particularly for beginners or those with certain health conditions. It's essential to choose a workout routine that fits your current fitness level, health status, and, most importantly, one that you enjoy. After all, the best workout for you is the one that you can sustain in the long term.

In addition, variety in your workout routine can be beneficial. It can help prevent boredom, reduce the risk of overuse injuries, and ensure a well-rounded fitness regimen.

Remember, the path to wellness does not lie in extremes but in balance. Engaging in a variety of physical activities that you enjoy is likely to be much more beneficial for your overall wellness than sticking to one type of high-intensity workout.

#4 Age or Physical Limitations Restrict Fitness

The belief that age or physical limitations restrict fitness is another pervasive myth. Many people think that they're too old to start a fitness program or that their physical limitations prevent them from exercising. However, this is a flawed perspective.

Fitness is not limited to a specific age group or to people without physical limitations. Everyone can benefit from an appropriate amount and type of physical activity. It's never too late to start, and there are countless ways to adapt exercises to suit individual abilities and needs.

As we age, exercise becomes even more important. It can help maintain strength and flexibility, boost mood, improve cognitive function, manage or prevent diseases, and improve quality of life. Similarly, for people with physical limitations, regular physical activity can aid in managing symptoms, improving mobility, and enhancing overall health and well-being.

The key is to find a type of exercise you enjoy and that suits your individual circumstances. This might mean seeking advice from a healthcare provider or fitness professional to ensure that the activity is safe and effective for you. Remember, the goal is not to compare yourself with others but to improve your own health and fitness, no matter where you're starting from.

#5 Wellness Is Only for the Affluent

The belief that wellness is only for the affluent is a misconception that often restricts people from making healthy lifestyle choices. It's easy to think that wellness requires expensive gym memberships, high-end workout gear, organic food, and other costly products and services. However, this isn't the case.

Wellness is not about how much you spend; it's about how you live. It's about making healthy choices, staying active, taking care of your mental health, building strong relationships, and finding purpose and satisfaction in life. None of these things requires a hefty bank balance.

Physical activity can be free. Walking, running, cycling, and bodyweight exercises are just a few examples of activities that don't cost anything. As for healthy eating, it's about choosing whole, unprocessed foods and planning meals ahead of time rather than opting for pricey 'superfoods' or organic labels.

Furthermore, practices such as mindfulness, meditation, and getting enough sleep - crucial aspects of holistic wellness - are free and accessible to everyone.

In short, wellness is not a luxury; it's a way of life. It's about making the most of what you have to enhance your health and happiness. Everyone, regardless of their financial status, has the right to wellness.

Now that we understand the concept of holistic wellness and have dispelled some misconceptions, let's delve into practical ways to incorporate it into our daily lives. In the upcoming chapter, we will explore the incorporation of holistic wellness and embark on a journey towards comprehensive well-being.

"Your past is not a blueprint for your future. You possess the strength to forge a fresh start."

– Kapil Mehrotra

Chapter - 4

The Happiness Blueprint: Striking a Balance

If holistic wellness is our ultimate destination, then the conscious choices we make in our everyday lives are the stepping stones leading us there. As we navigate through the myriad responsibilities, commitments, and desires that colour our existence, striking a balance can seem like a daunting task. However, finding this equilibrium is the key to sustainable wellness and contentment.

Mastering Time Management: Tips and Tricks

Time, the invisible river that we all flow with, is an entity that remains constant, no matter where we stand in life. Each day, every person is gifted with the same 24 hours, a precious and limited resource that we cannot store or purchase. And for the ambitious urban Indian, who aspires to strike a balance between their personal and professional lives while making room for a fitness routine, the art of time management is not just a skill but a necessity.

Living in a fast-paced world, it often feels as if there are not enough hours in a day to get everything done. From meeting work deadlines to family responsibilities, social commitments, and personal care, our lives are packed with endless tasks. Amidst this chaos, carving out time for fitness and wellness can seem like a Herculean task.

Yet, in reality, time management is less about scrambling to get more done and more about organizing and controlling your time to focus on your priorities, including your health and well-being. It is about making smart decisions that align with your wellness goals.

So, how can one navigate the choppy waters of time management? The answer lies in two critical strategies: prioritizing tasks and leveraging technology. By understanding and implementing these, one can not only create more time but also utilize it effectively, ensuring holistic wellness isn't compromised.

Let us delve into each of these strategies, unravelling how they can be harnessed to create harmony between our daily routines and the pursuit of holistic wellness.

Prioritizing Tasks: Essential vs. Non-Essential

The idea of task prioritization may not be new to you, but applying it consciously in your life, with a specific focus on promoting wellness, can have profound implications. The term 'essential' is highly personal and reflects activities that significantly impact your life quality, align with your values, and contribute to your overall wellness. On the other hand, 'non-essential' tasks are those which may seem pressing at the moment but have minimal or no impact on your life's larger narrative, your growth, and your wellness.

Often, we find ourselves consumed by tasks that appear urgent but are, in reality, not important in our life's grand scheme. By redefining our boundaries and asserting control over how we choose to spend our time, we free up mental and physical space to focus on activities that contribute to our holistic wellness.

For instance, spending quality time with loved ones, practising self-care, learning a new skill, or engaging in physical activity can be labelled as 'essential,' as they contribute significantly to our physical, emotional, and mental well-being. In contrast, spending excessive time on work beyond office hours, compulsive usage of social media, or getting embroiled in unnecessary disputes can be considered 'non-essential' tasks as they drain energy and detract from our wellness.

Recognizing the essential from the non-essential is not an overnight process. It requires reflection and honest self-assessment. It may involve tough choices, like cutting back on late-night television to ensure a good night's sleep or resisting the urge to check emails while spending time with family.

However, it's crucial to remember that this process isn't about achieving perfection. It's about progression and making small yet consistent choices that reflect your commitment to wellness. So, as you move ahead in this journey, let the mantra of 'essential versus non-essential' guide you towards greater control over your time and a more balanced and fulfilling life.

Leveraging Technology: Utilizing Apps and Tools for Productivity

In the era of fast-paced living and digital innovations, the use of technology has become an inevitable part of our lives. It's not an understatement to say that technology has its fingerprints on almost every aspect of our daily routine. From communication to entertainment, and from shopping to learning – it's all just a click away. But can technology contribute to our wellness journey? Absolutely, if used judiciously.

Technology can either be a roadblock or a facilitator on your path to holistic wellness, depending on how you use it. Let's shift our perspective and look at technology as an enabler that can help you manage time and resources effectively.

Productivity tools and apps offer one of the most convenient ways to organize your life. Take, for example, task management apps like Google Keep, Todoist, or Evernote. These platforms can help you create and manage to-do lists, set reminders, and delegate tasks, effectively helping you prioritize the 'essential' over the 'non-essential.'

Calendar apps such as Google Calendar or Microsoft Outlook not only assist you in planning your day, week, or even your month ahead but also provide features to set reminders for important events or deadlines. By effectively scheduling your tasks, you can avoid last-minute rushes and stress, leaving you with more time for self-care and wellness activities.

Moreover, there's a plethora of wellness-specific apps designed to guide you on the path to better health and fitness. Fitness trackers like Apple's Health, Google Fit, or Strava can help monitor your physical activities, set fitness goals, and track your progress. Diet and nutrition apps like HealthifyMe can guide your meal planning and help monitor your calorie intake. Mental wellness apps like Headspace or Calm can provide guided meditation sessions, sleep stories, or mindfulness exercises to help manage stress and anxiety.

But remember, the idea is not to become reliant on technology or to get lost in the sea of productivity or wellness apps. The goal is to judiciously choose tools that align with your lifestyle, personal preferences, and wellness goals. Let these digital enablers assist you in creating a routine that prioritizes wellness and facilitates a better work-life balance.

Embracing Flexibility: Adapting to Unexpected Changes in Schedule

When it comes to managing time and ensuring productivity, flexibility is not usually the first trait that comes to mind. We often imagine a rigid schedule, meticulously planned and adhered to, as the epitome of time management. But as with all aspects of life, unexpected events can disrupt even the most carefully planned schedules. Here's where flexibility comes into play.

The ability to adapt to unexpected changes in your schedule is a vital skill in the quest for holistic wellness. It's not about abandoning your plan at the first sign of disruption but finding ways to accommodate these unforeseen changes without compromising on your wellness goals.

Suppose an urgent work meeting encroaches upon your workout time. Instead of entirely skipping the workout, consider adjusting the intensity or duration to fit the reduced timeframe, or explore options to reschedule it later in the day. If a late-night project threatens your sleep schedule, consider compensating by taking short power naps during the day or ensuring you get enough rest the following day.

Flexibility also extends to your wellness routines. Variety, as they say, is the spice of life. Alternating between different types of physical exercises, trying out various mindful practices, or experimenting with diverse nutritious foods can not only keep your wellness journey exciting but also ensure a comprehensive and balanced approach to health.

Embracing flexibility doesn't mean being inconsistent. It's about building a robust yet adaptable plan that caters to the ebb and flow of life. As you continue to master this balance, you'll find it easier to navigate unexpected disruptions without letting them derail your wellness journey.

Living Authentically: Avoiding Comparison and Embracing Individuality

In the fast-paced world of today, it's easy to find ourselves lost in the whirlwind of comparison. Every social media notification serves as a reminder of someone else's accomplishments, their seemingly perfect lives playing out in vibrant pictures and captions. This constant influx of information feeds into our innate tendency to compare our lives with those of others. The immediate gratification that comes from a well-liked post or an admired picture creates an illusion of success that is hard to compete with. This is what we refer to as the 'comparison trap'.

The comparison trap is a formidable obstacle in our pursuit of authenticity and holistic wellness. When we measure our lives against the highlight reels of others, we create unrealistic expectations for ourselves. We forget that each individual's journey is different, filled with unique triumphs and setbacks. We overlook the fact that what's portrayed online is often a distorted reflection of reality, carefully curated to showcase the best moments while concealing the struggles.

Falling into this trap can lead to a host of negative emotions, including feelings of inadequacy, discontentment, and stress. It can undermine our self-confidence and lead us to question our self-worth. The joy of our own achievements may be overshadowed by the success of others. Consequently, this constant comparison can derail our wellness journey, diverting our focus from personal growth to competition.

However, once we understand the implications of the comparison trap, we can start to disengage from it. It requires conscious effort to redirect our focus from others' lives to our own, to appreciate our unique journey, and to define success on our own terms. In the upcoming sections, we will explore practical strategies to break free from the comparison trap, fostering a healthier relationship with ourselves and our social media platforms.

Remember, comparison may be the thief of joy, but authenticity is the key to wellness. It's time to step away from the illusions cast by others' lives and to start embracing our unique path towards holistic wellness.

Embracing Individuality: Celebrating Uniqueness

In a world that often seeks conformity, embracing individuality is a brave and rewarding journey. Your path to holistic wellness is not about fitting into a specific mould or meeting a generalized standard of health. Instead, it is about celebrating your unique characteristics, your strengths, your weaknesses, and even your quirks. It's about understanding that your wellness journey is just that - yours.

The importance of individuality in the pursuit of wellness cannot be overstated. Everyone has a unique body composition, metabolic rate, lifestyle, and preferences, which means that a one-size-fits-all approach to wellness seldom works. Instead, embracing your individuality can help tailor a wellness regime that suits you, one that takes into account your personal circumstances, preferences, and goals.

Embracing individuality goes beyond just the physical aspects of wellness. It encompasses mental and emotional well-being too. Understanding and accepting your emotional responses, managing stress in a way that works for you, and practising self-care activities that you genuinely enjoy, are all part of living authentically.

Set personal goals that align with your lifestyle and aspirations. Measure your success not against others, but against your own progress. Remember, wellness is not a race or a competition. It is a journey, one that is meant to enhance your life, not add to its pressures.

Tips for Setting SMART Goals:

Author, Brian Tracy's influential work 'Goals', illuminates the transformative power of structured goal setting in the pursuit of personal success and fulfilment. Tracy opines that by delineating a distinct pathway for our ambitions, we empower ourselves to focus on our personal objectives, thereby reducing the pull of unhealthy comparison.

Tracy underscores the concept of setting SMART (Specific, Measurable, Achievable, Relevant, and Time-bound) goals. This approach ensures our health objectives are not only realistic but are also within our reach. By segmenting our fitness aspirations into smaller, manageable increments, we can foster motivation and progressively move towards our wellness targets.

Let's deconstruct the SMART goal-setting framework in the context of fitness and provide an illustrative example:

- **Specific:** A specific fitness goal is detailed and distinct, pinpointing exactly what health outcome you are aiming for. This enhances focus and directs your energy and effort towards the achievement of this goal.

- *Example: A generic fitness goal like "I want to be healthier," can be made specific by stating, "I want to be able to run 5 kilometres."*

- **Measurable:** A measurable fitness goal incorporates quantifiable indicators to track your progress. It helps keep you inspired, and if needed, facilitates strategic modifications to ensure you're on track.

  Example: If your specific goal is to run 5 kilometres, the measurable component could be the distance you run each week, allowing you to chart your improvement.

- **Achievable:** An achievable fitness goal is one that takes into account your current physical condition, resources, and constraints. It should be challenging enough to incite action but not so difficult that it appears unreachable, leading to demotivation.

  Example: If you're new to running, aiming to complete a full marathon in a month may not be achievable. However, working towards running a 5K in three months might be a realistic and achievable goal.

- **Relevant:** A relevant fitness goal is one that aligns with your broader wellness objectives and personal values. This ensures the goal is meaningful and worth pursuing, keeping you engaged and committed to the process.

  Example: If your overarching goal is to boost your stamina and physical endurance, running a 5K could be a relevant fitness objective contributing to this larger ambition.

- **Time-bound:** A time-bound fitness goal features a specific end date. This creates a sense of urgency, fosters prioritization, and discourages procrastination, thereby enhancing accountability.

Example: To make the goal of running 5 kilometres time-bound, you could commit to accomplishing this within three months.

So, a SMART fitness goal could be: "I aim to run 5 kilometres within the next three months by training for 30 minutes, five times a week, and maintaining a balanced diet."

Striking a balance in life is an art that can be mastered with conscious effort, careful planning, and consistent practice. This balance goes beyond merely juggling responsibilities or ticking off tasks on a to-do list. It is about aligning your daily routines with the principles of holistic wellness, prioritizing your health and well-being, and ensuring they are not sidelined in the pursuit of professional success or social obligations.

Your wellness is in your hands. It is a choice you make every day, in every task you undertake, in every decision you make.

"People may blame and criticize you. Don't respond in kind. Instead, focus on self-improvement and success to prove them wrong."

– Kapil Mehrotra

Chapter - 5

You Against the World: Starting the Fitness Journey

Having gained a solid understanding of how to prioritize, leverage technology, and embrace flexibility, we are now well-prepared to embark on our personal fitness journey. While the road ahead might appear challenging, it's important to remember that "every journey begins with a single step." There's no better way to start this journey than by crafting a comprehensive fitness plan.

Creating a 21-Day Fitness Plan

The concept of a 21-day fitness plan is built around the notion that it takes 21 days to form a new habit or break an old one. This idea stems from Dr. Maxwell Maltz's observations in the 1960s where he noticed that amputees took, on average, 21 days to adjust to the loss of a limb. His findings led to the popularization of the "21-day rule" in the field of self-help and behaviour modification.

While more recent research suggests that the time to form a new habit may vary depending on the complexity of the behaviour and the individual, the 21-day rule continues to provide a solid framework for setting and achieving short-term goals. This time period is long enough to see meaningful progress but short enough to maintain motivation and focus.

In the context of fitness, adopting a 21-day plan can create momentum and establish consistent exercise and dietary habits. It serves as a solid starting point for those who are beginning their fitness journey or looking to break through a plateau. Over the course of these three weeks, you're not just working towards physical improvement, but you're also conditioning your mind to accept this new routine as part of your lifestyle. The ultimate goal is to transform these actions from 'tasks that need to be done' into 'behaviours that happen automatically.'

Let's align the SMART goal framework discussed in the previous chapter to your 21-day fitness plan. SMART goals are goals that are Specific, Measurable, Attainable, Relevant, and Time-bound. Each of these characteristics can give your fitness plan the structure and direction it needs to be effective.

Once you define your SMART goal, the next step is to map out how they fit into your 21-day fitness plan. Here's how each aspect can be incorporated:

Specific - Identify specific exercises, dietary changes, and other actions that will help you achieve each of your fitness goals.

Measurable - Determine how you'll track your progress towards each goal throughout the 21 days. This could involve monitoring your workout durations, tracking the weights you lift, recording the distances you run or cycle, or keeping a food diary.

Attainable - Ensure your fitness plan is realistic given your current fitness level and other commitments. For example, if your goal is to run 5km, your plan might start with short, manageable runs, gradually increasing in distance.

Relevant - Make sure each element of your fitness plan relates back to your broader goals. If you're aiming to improve cardiovascular fitness, your plan should incorporate cardio exercises. If you're looking to gain strength, weightlifting or resistance training should be included.

Time-bound - Use the 21-day framework as your time-bound aspect. By having a clear start and end date, you can stay focused and motivated.

This approach takes you one step closer to turning your fitness goals into a lifestyle, moving beyond just the initial three weeks.

Day-by-Day Approach: Breaking Down Activities and Targets

Once you've aligned your 21-day fitness plan with your SMART goals, the next step is to break down your activities and targets on a day-by-day basis. Having a daily plan not only organizes your fitness journey but also aids in maintaining consistency, which is vital for habit formation.

Here's how you can approach the day-by-day planning of your 21-day fitness journey:

- *Decide the Focus for Each Day* - Start by outlining the focus of each day. Depending on your goals, this might be cardio, strength training, flexibility exercises, or rest and recovery. It's crucial to incorporate a variety of exercise types into your week to promote balanced physical development and prevent overuse injuries.

- *Set Daily Targets* – For each day, set a specific target that aligns with your broader goals. For instance, if your focus is cardio, your target might be to run for a certain amount of time or distance.

- *Plan Your Routine* – With your focus and target in mind, plan your specific routine for each day. This might include specific exercises, sets, and repetitions for strength training or certain routes and paces for cardio.

- *Consider Rest and Recovery* – Rest and recovery are as important as the workouts themselves. Ensure that you include rest days in your plan, and consider lighter, active recovery days where you engage in low-intensity activities like walking or yoga.

- *Remember Nutrition* – Consider your nutrition plan for each day, ensuring it aligns with your activity level. For instance, on heavy workout days, you might need more calories and protein to fuel your body and aid recovery.

- *Be Open to Adjustment* – Finally, remember that it's okay to adjust your plan as you progress. If you find a certain workout too challenging or not challenging enough, tweak your plan accordingly. Listen to your body and make changes as necessary.

Exercise Selection: Combining Cardio, Strength, and Flexibility Training

Once your daily activities and targets have been set, it's time to delve into the specifics of the exercise routines that will help you reach your fitness objectives. Your fitness plan should include a combination of cardio, strength, and flexibility exercises, each with unique benefits that contribute to your overall health and wellness.

- *Cardiovascular Exercises* - Cardio exercises are essential for improving heart health, boosting lung capacity, and burning calories. This category of exercise includes activities like running, swimming, biking, or even brisk walking. These can be tailored according to your fitness level. For instance, a beginner might start with brisk walks, gradually incorporating running intervals, and eventually progressing to full runs.

- *Strength Training* - Strength training exercises help in building muscle mass, improving bone density, and boosting metabolism. These exercises can involve weightlifting, bodyweight exercises like push-ups and squats, or resistance band workouts. Similar to cardio, strength training should be progressive. Beginners might start with bodyweight exercises and gradually incorporate weights as they build strength.

- *Flexibility Training* - Flexibility exercises are often overlooked but are crucial in maintaining a full range of motion in the joints, reducing the risk of injuries, and aiding recovery. These exercises often involve stretching and can be incorporated into your warm-up and cool-down routines. Activities like yoga and Pilates also improve flexibility while providing additional benefits like improved core strength and stress reduction.

When selecting your exercises, it's crucial to keep variety in mind. Varying your workouts not only promotes a more balanced physical development but also helps to keep your workouts interesting and exciting, increasing the likelihood of adherence to your fitness plan.

A Sample Workout Plan

Here's a sample workout chart if you are just getting started:

Week 1

- Day 1: (Cardio) 20-minute brisk walking + 5-minute cooldown stretch

- Day 2: (Strength) Bodyweight exercises - 3 sets of 10 squats, push-ups, and lunges each

- Day 3: (Cardio) 25-minute brisk walking + 5-minute cooldown stretch

- Day 4: (Strength) Same as Day 2, add planks - 3 sets of 30 seconds each

- Day 5: (Cardio) Introduce a 5-minute slow jog within the 30-minute session

- Day 6 and 7: (Recovery) 30-minute yoga or stretching routine

Week 2

- Day 8: (Cardio) Increase jogging to 10 minutes within the 30-minute session

- Day 9: (Strength) Same as Day 4, add dumbbell curls and shoulder presses if available

- Day 10: (Cardio) 15-minute jogging + 15-minute brisk walk

- Day 11: (Strength) Add one more set to each exercise from Day 9

- Day 12: (Cardio) Try to jog for 20 minutes continuously

- Day 13 and 14: (Recovery) Add a gentle cycle ride or swim to your recovery routine if possible

Week 3

- Day 15: (Cardio) Aim for 25-minute continuous jogging

- Day 16: (Strength) Further increase the reps of each exercise, if possible

- Day 17: (Cardio) Try to reach the 30-minute continuous jogging goal

- Day 18: (Strength) Add more complex exercises like burpees or deadlifts if feasible

- Day 19: (Cardio) Maintain the 30-minute continuous jogging

- Day 20 and 21: (Recovery) A full-body massage session to reward yourself for the hard work

A Sample Dietary Plan

Breakfast:

- Option 1: A bowl of poha with added veggies and a sprinkle of peanuts for some protein.

- Option 2: Moong dal chilla (savoury pancakes) with green chutney.

Mid-Morning Snack:

- A small bowl of mixed sprouts or a piece of fresh fruit.

Lunch:

- A balanced thali comprising of roti (whole wheat if possible), a portion of dal for protein, a serving of seasonal sabzi (vegetable dish), and some curd. Include a side salad for extra fibre and micronutrients.

Afternoon Snack:

- A small bowl of roasted chickpeas or murmura (puffed rice) mix.

Dinner:

- A lighter meal like khichdi (made from rice and lentils) with a side of mixed vegetable raita.

Before Bed:

- A glass of warm milk, if desired Golden (Turmeric) Milk

Please note, the focus should still be on portion control and balance - getting a mix of protein, fibre, healthy fats, and carbohydrates in each meal. Be mindful of the oil used in cooking and aim to have a variety of fruits and vegetables throughout the day to ensure a mix of different nutrients.

Disclaimer : The above suggestions are generic of workouts and diets; they change if you have any existing comorbidities or medical issues.

"Strive not for perfection but for progress, aiming to be better today than you were yesterday."

– Kapil Mehrotra

Chapter - 6

Unleashing Your Inner Fire: Maintaining Motivation

Motivation is like a car's engine - it's what gets you moving. In terms of fitness, it's that little voice in your head that says "Let's do this!" when you'd rather sit on the couch. But where does this 'get-up-and-go' come from? Well, there are two main fuel sources: intrinsic and extrinsic motivation.

Intrinsic motivation is all about doing something because it makes you feel good inside. It's that warm, fuzzy feeling you get when you've smashed your personal best or when you've been consistent with your fitness plan for a whole week. This kind of motivation comes from within and tends to stick around for the long haul because it's tied to personal satisfaction and joy.

Extrinsic motivation, on the flip side, is sparked by outside factors. It might be the desire to look fantastic for your best friend's wedding, the urge to keep up with your competitive cousin at the next family 5K run, or even the wish to fit into societal beauty standards. These are powerful motivators, sure, but they might flicker out once the wedding is over, the race is run, or the trends change.

The key here is to understand what fuels your fitness engine. Is it an inside job? Or do you need a bit of an outside push? Recognizing what drives you can help you keep that fitness fire blazing, whether you're on day 1 or day 21 of your fitness plan.

The Psychology of Motivation: A Look into the Human Mind

Peeking into the human mind, motivation isn't just a simple trigger-and-response mechanism. It's far more complex and deeply intertwined with our psychology. From a psychological perspective, motivation can be influenced by our needs, desires, fears, and even our self-image.

For instance, Maslow's Hierarchy of Needs, a famous psychological theory, suggests that our actions are motivated by our unmet needs. When applied to fitness, this could mean that someone might start working out to fulfil a basic need (like health) or a psychological need (like esteem or self-confidence).

Another psychological aspect is the Fear of Missing Out (FOMO). Seeing others achieve their fitness goals, especially in today's social media era, can create a desire to be part of the 'fit community.' This social motivation can be a powerful push towards starting and maintaining a fitness routine.

Lastly, our self-image, the way we perceive ourselves, can significantly influence our motivation. If we view ourselves as active and healthy individuals, we're more likely to be motivated to engage in fitness activities.

Understanding these psychological aspects can provide valuable insights into our own motivation, allowing us to tap into these triggers when our fitness fire starts to dwindle.

Setting and Implementing Fitness Goals: The First Step Towards Motivation

The commencement of any fitness journey revolves around setting defined and precise goals. This acts as a compass, guiding our actions and helping maintain our motivation. Whether it's shedding a few pounds, running a marathon, or simply being able to do a set of push-ups, having a clear goal is critical.

Without a goal, our efforts may become aimless, leading to dejection and decreased motivation over time. On the other hand, setting a challenging yet achievable goal can create a sense of excitement and anticipation, providing the initial burst of motivation to kickstart our fitness journey.

But how does one go about setting effective fitness goals? The key lies in the SMART framework we discussed in the previous chapters. Your goals should be Specific, Measurable, Achievable, Relevant, and Time-bound. For instance, instead of setting a vague goal like 'I want to get fit,' opt for something more specific like 'I want to lose 10 pounds in the next three months.'

Setting SMART goals is not just about being clear about the 'what' but also understanding the 'why.' Reflecting on the reasons behind your goal - whether it's feeling healthier, looking better, or increasing your lifespan - can enhance your emotional connection with your goal, providing an additional boost to your motivation.

Consistency is key when it comes to fitness. In fact, it is one of the main pillars that holds the structure of your fitness journey. A consistent fitness routine helps you establish discipline, creates a sense of achievement, and builds your motivation over time.

The first step to creating consistency is to schedule your workouts. Find a time in the day that you can consistently devote to exercise. Make sure to consider your daily responsibilities and energy levels throughout the day to find the best fit. Your workout schedule should not feel like a burden; instead, it should be a positive and invigorating part of your day.

Another effective strategy to maintain motivation in your fitness journey is to leverage support systems around you. This could be friends, family, or fitness communities that share the same fitness goals.

Working out with friends or family can make the experience more enjoyable and less of a chore. It can also foster a sense of friendly competition, which can push you to perform better. Moreover, having someone who understands your journey and can provide support during tough times can make a huge difference in keeping your motivation high.

Fitness communities, both offline and online, can also be a great source of motivation. These communities are often filled with people who are on a similar journey, offering a platform to share experiences, advice, and encouragement. They can provide a sense of belonging and a space to celebrate your achievements.

The more consistent you are, the quicker you'll see progress, and progress is one of the greatest motivators. Whether it's muscle growth, weight loss, or improved endurance, visible improvements serve as affirmations of your efforts and fuel your motivation to push further.

Moreover, consistency helps in developing self-discipline, which can come in handy during times when your motivation is running low. There will be days when you don't feel like working out or eating healthy but having developed the habit of consistency, you'll be more likely to stick to your routine.

Embracing Failure: Understanding and Learning from Mistakes

Everyone experiences failure at some point in their fitness journey. It's a universal truth that can be hard to accept. However, the first step to overcoming failure is to embrace it. Accepting that mistakes and setbacks are not the end, but rather a part of the journey is critical.

Failure is nothing more than feedback - it tells you where you went wrong and what you need to correct. Instead of viewing failure as a negative outcome, see it as an opportunity to learn and grow. By analyzing your mistakes, you can identify the areas you need to work on and devise strategies to improve them.

Furthermore, remember that failure is not unique to you. Every successful person in the world, whether in fitness or any other field, has experienced failure. What sets them apart is their ability to turn their failures into stepping stones towards success. So, next time you stumble, don't be disheartened. Stand back up, dust yourself off, learn from your mistake, and move forward.

There's a popular saying that goes, "The only constant in life is change," and this absolutely holds in the realm of fitness. As you journey on the path of physical well-being, you'll encounter various obstacles that might hinder your progress. Some days, you might feel like you're not making progress or have hit a stagnation point. It's during these challenging times that your willpower will be put to the test.

Here are some strategies you can employ to navigate through such obstacles:

- **Change Your Routine:** One common reason for hitting a plateau is that our bodies have adapted to our routines. The solution is to introduce changes – vary the intensity, duration, or type of exercises you are doing. If you're used to jogging, try cycling or swimming. If you've been doing weight lifting, add yoga or pilates to your regimen. This can kick-start your body into a new growth phase.

- **Revisit Your Goals:** Sometimes, stagnation is a result of vague or unrealistic goals. Take a step back and reevaluate your objectives. Are they SMART (Specific, Measurable, Achievable, Relevant, and Time-bound)? If not, redefine them.

- **Seek Support:** Connect with a support group, be it a fitness club, an online community, or a personal trainer. Sharing your experiences with others who are on the same journey can give you a fresh perspective, renewed inspiration, and practical tips to overcome your hurdles.

- **Mind Over Matter:** Cultivate a positive mindset. Practice mindfulness and self-compassion. Understand that progress isn't always linear and that setbacks are part of the journey. Use affirmations and visualizations to maintain a positive and motivated frame of mind.

- **Nutrition Check:** If you're experiencing physical stagnation, your diet might be the culprit. Ensure you're consuming a balanced diet rich in proteins, carbs, and healthy fats. You may want to consult a nutritionist to tailor a dietary plan that suits your fitness goals.

Remember, obstacles and stagnation phases are not roadblocks but stepping stones towards your goal. They challenge you to step out of your comfort zone, test your commitment, and eventually make you stronger.

Rekindling Motivation: Tips for Reigniting Your Fitness Passion

Every fitness journey can have its highs and lows. Sometimes, the flame of motivation that once burned so brightly might start to flicker. During such times, it's essential to have a set of strategies in your toolbox to reignite your passion for fitness. Here's how you can stoke the fire of motivation and keep it blazing:

- **Rediscover Your 'Why':** What inspired you to start this fitness journey in the first place? Revisiting your original goals and reasons can help rekindle that initial passion. Write them down and keep them somewhere you can see them every day to serve as a constant reminder.

- **Try New Activities:** If your usual workout has started to feel like a chore, mix things up. Try a new sport, a different fitness class, or a novel exercise routine. New experiences can help renew your excitement and enthusiasm.

- **Celebrate Small Wins:** Progress can be slow, and the big goals can seem far off. However, celebrating small victories along the way can boost your motivation. Did you work out five days in a row? Did you lift heavier weights this week? Acknowledge and celebrate these achievements!

- **Connect with Inspiring People:** Surround yourself with people who inspire you. This could be a workout buddy, a fitness role model you follow online, or even a personal trainer. Their energy and drive can spark your own motivation.

- **Reflect and Recharge:** Sometimes, a dip in motivation might be a sign that you need a break. It's okay to take some time off to rest and recharge. Use this time to reflect on your journey so far and visualize the progress you want to make moving forward.

Remember, motivation is not a fixed entity – it ebbs and flows. But with the right mindset and strategies, you can keep it burning strong and continue pushing forward on your fitness journey.

"The difference between a successful person and others is not a lack of strength, not a lack of knowledge, but rather a lack in will."

– Vince Lombardi

Chapter - 7

Understanding the Connection Between Physical and Mental Health

Just as our bodies influence our minds, our minds can significantly impact our bodies. This intricate, two-way interaction is a cornerstone of holistic fitness, which goes beyond the mere physical aspects to delve into mental and emotional realms.

The crossroads of physical health and mental health form a bustling junction. Each influences the other in numerous, often surprising, ways. For instance, regular exercise triggers the release of endorphins—your body's natural mood elevators. They help decrease stress levels, alleviate anxiety, boost self-esteem, and even enhance sleep quality.

Engaging in physical activity can also serve as a form of meditation, allowing you to lose yourself in the rhythm of repetitive movements—an escape from the constant mental chatter. As a result, you may experience a heightened sense of awareness, clarity, and focus in your day-to-day life.

Inversely, if you're physically inactive, you're more likely to experience depression or anxiety. Chronic physical conditions, such as heart disease or diabetes, can also contribute to mental health disorders, highlighting the symbiotic relationship between physical and mental health.

Emotional Resilience: The Impact of Mental Health on Physical Well-being

As we delve further into the connection between mental and physical health, the concept of emotional resilience plays a key role. Emotional resilience refers to one's ability to adapt to stressful situations or crises. More resilient individuals can 'bounce back' from adversity and move forward, potentially strengthening their mental well-being in the process.

Mental health issues such as stress, anxiety, or depression can adversely affect your physical health. For instance, chronic stress can lead to conditions like heart disease, high blood pressure, and weakened immune function. Anxiety disorders can cause digestive or bowel problems, like irritable bowel syndrome. Depression not only induces lethargy and reduces the motivation to stay active but it's also linked to chronic illnesses like diabetes and obesity.

However, having robust emotional resilience can act as a protective shield against these potential health problems. By managing stress levels and maintaining a positive outlook, resilient individuals may reduce the negative physical impacts of mental health issues. They are often better equipped to maintain a regular exercise routine, make healthier food choices, and prioritize sleep— all critical components of physical health.

Developing emotional resilience often involves strategies like cognitive-behavioural therapy, mindfulness meditation, stress management techniques, and fostering strong social relationships. It's worth noting that emotional resilience doesn't mean avoiding or suppressing negative emotions. Instead, it's about understanding and accepting these emotions and learning how to manage them effectively.

Emotional resilience, like any other skill, can be developed and strengthened over time. It is not an inherent trait that only some 'lucky' individuals possess. This realization opens a world of possibilities, where each one of us can cultivate and improve our emotional resilience to benefit both our mental and physical health.

Working on emotional resilience is much like training for physical strength. Just as you would start lifting lighter weights and gradually move on to heavier ones, building emotional resilience begins with managing smaller stressors and eventually handling major life crises. And similar to the soreness you feel after a rigorous workout, the process may be uncomfortable. Yet, it's this very discomfort that fosters growth and resilience.

Here are a few ways you can enhance your emotional resilience:

1. Practice Mindfulness: Mindfulness is about staying in the present moment, without judgment. Regular practice can help you manage stress, reduce negative emotions, and improve overall mental well-being. This can range from formal mindfulness meditation practices to simply staying focused during everyday activities like washing dishes or walking.

2. Nurture Positive Relationships: Building strong, positive relationships and social connections can provide emotional support during tough times. Sharing your feelings with someone you trust can alleviate stress and provide a fresh perspective on challenging situations.

3. Embrace Self-Care: Prioritize activities that you enjoy and that help you relax. This could be reading a book, going for a walk, listening to your favourite music, or anything else that helps you unwind. Regular self-care can help recharge your emotional batteries and increase resilience.

4. Positive Affirmations and Self-Talk: The way you talk to yourself matters. Cultivate a habit of positive self-talk and use affirmations to foster a positive mindset. This can help you navigate through life's ups and downs with a more optimistic outlook.

5. Professional Help: Don't hesitate to seek professional help if you feel overwhelmed. Psychologists and therapists can provide tools and techniques to build emotional resilience and improve mental health.

By incorporating these strategies into your life, you can bolster your emotional resilience, providing a strong foundation for both your mental and physical health.

Scientific Evidence: Studies Linking Physical Fitness and Mental Health

The intersection of physical fitness and mental health is a vibrant field of scientific research, with numerous studies underscoring their intertwined relationship. Let's dive into some of the compelling evidence that connects the dots between these two crucial aspects of human health.

Exercise and Depression: A seminal study published in the Journal of Psychiatric Practice makes a compelling case for the therapeutic potential of regular physical exercise in combating depression. This research suggests that for some individuals, exercise can serve as an effective alternative to traditional depression treatments, such as medication or psychotherapy.

Depression, a mental health disorder characterized by persistent feelings of sadness and disinterest, can significantly hamper an individual's quality of life. Conventional treatments typically involve antidepressants, cognitive-behavioural therapy (CBT), or a combination of both. While these methods can be effective, they're not universally so, and some individuals may struggle with side effects or lack of progress.

This is where exercise steps in as a promising complementary or even alternative treatment option. Physical activity spurs the release of endorphins, often dubbed as 'feel-good' hormones, due to their ability to produce feelings of euphoria and general well-being. Exercise also encourages the production of serotonin and norepinephrine, neurotransmitters that play a pivotal role in mood regulation.

What makes the study's findings even more remarkable is the suggested potential of exercise to prevent relapses into depression. The relapsing nature of depression makes it a challenging disorder to handle, with many individuals experiencing multiple episodes throughout their lives. Regular exercise, according to the study, can act as a protective factor, reducing the likelihood of future depressive episodes.

Exercise, therefore, offers a two-pronged approach - it can alleviate current depressive symptoms and build resilience against future episodes. It's crucial, however, to remember that the effectiveness of exercise as a treatment may vary from person to person and shouldn't replace professional help. Always consult with a healthcare professional when considering treatment options for depression.

Physical Activity and Anxiety: An enlightening article in the American Journal of Psychiatry presents a notable correlation between physical inactivity and anxiety disorders. Anxiety disorders, which encompass a wide range of conditions such as generalized anxiety disorder, panic disorder, and social anxiety disorder, are characterized by excessive worry, feelings of dread, and physical symptoms like a rapid heartbeat or restlessness. These disorders can significantly impact an individual's ability to lead a fulfilling life.

The study suggests that those who lead a sedentary lifestyle are more prone to experience these symptoms, hinting at the negative mental health effects of physical inactivity. On the flip side, the article posits that incorporating regular physical activity into one's routine can alleviate symptoms of anxiety, ultimately fostering a sense of well-being.

This positive correlation between exercise and reduced anxiety symptoms stems from various physiological and psychological mechanisms. On a biological level, engaging in physical activity stimulates the release of endorphins, serotonin, and other neurochemicals that act as natural mood stabilizers. Additionally, exercise can act as a distraction from worrying thoughts, allowing individuals to break the cycle of negative rumination that often accompanies anxiety disorders.

Moreover, physical activity provides individuals with a sense of accomplishment. Each workout completed or fitness goal achieved can boost self-efficacy and self-esteem, key factors in fostering mental resilience. Over time, this sense of mastery and progress can help individuals better manage their anxiety symptoms, increasing their confidence in their ability to cope with stressful situations.

The research strongly points to regular physical activity as a potentially powerful tool in the arsenal against anxiety disorders. However, as with depression, it's essential to note that while exercise can be an effective supplementary intervention, it shouldn't replace professional medical treatment. The approach to managing anxiety should be multi-faceted, encompassing professional help, possibly medication, psychotherapy, lifestyle changes, and, yes, regular physical exercise.

Exercise and Brain Health: A ground-breaking research study published in the Journal of Clinical Psychology demonstrates a compelling link between physical exercise and the health of our brains. It shows that engaging in physical activity stimulates the production of a protein known as brain-derived neurotrophic factor (BDNF). This protein is a key player in the growth, maintenance, and survival of neurons - the building blocks of the brain.

BDNF is often likened to fertilizer for the brain because of its role in facilitating brain plasticity, which is the brain's capacity to reorganize itself, adapt to new information, and form new memories. This means that when you exercise and your heart rate increases, you're not only strengthening your heart and muscles but also enhancing your brain's potential for growth and development.

The implications of this are profound. Higher levels of BDNF are associated with improved cognitive function, including better memory, attention, and processing speed. This is particularly important as we age and naturally experience a decline in these cognitive functions. Regular physical activity could, therefore, play a pivotal role in protecting against cognitive decline and neurodegenerative diseases such as Alzheimer's and Parkinson's.

Furthermore, BDNF has been found to have a protective effect against mental health conditions like depression and anxiety. This aligns with the earlier discussions on the positive impact of exercise on these conditions, further solidifying the connection between physical activity and mental well-being.

However, it's crucial to bear in mind that while exercise can significantly boost brain health, it is just one piece of the puzzle. A balanced diet, sufficient sleep, mental stimulation, and social interaction all contribute to maintaining a healthy brain.

Fitness and Self-Esteem: A comprehensive review of multiple studies, as published in Sports Medicine, puts forth a compelling argument for the positive relationship between physical activity and self-esteem, especially amongst children and adolescents. But the effect is not limited to these age groups; adults, too, can reap the benefits of this positive relationship.

When individuals engage in regular physical activity, it's not just their body that changes. Their perception of themselves and their bodies often changes too. As individuals work out and begin to observe improvements in their strength, flexibility, endurance, and perhaps even changes in their body composition, their self-confidence can start to rise. This boost in confidence extends beyond physical attributes, seeping into their perception of their capabilities and their sense of self-worth, thus elevating their overall self-esteem.

The relationship between exercise and self-esteem is reciprocal. As individuals feel better about themselves, they are more likely to continue participating in physical activity, which in turn continues to boost their self-esteem. It's a positive cycle that promotes both physical and mental well-being.

Improvement in body image is another key factor linking physical fitness and self-esteem. Regular exercise can lead to a greater appreciation for one's body, not just for how it looks, but more importantly, for what it can do. This shift in focus from appearance to performance can lead to a healthier and more positive body image.

Moreover, the sense of accomplishment that comes from achieving fitness goals, however small they may be, can also contribute significantly to self-esteem. Every personal record broken, every extra mile run, and every additional weight lifted serves as evidence of one's capabilities, reinforcing a positive self-concept.

However, it's important to approach fitness with the right mindset to foster a positive relationship with self-esteem. Setting realistic goals, celebrating progress, and avoiding comparison with others are vital for a healthy fitness journey that boosts self-esteem.

Exercise and Sleep: A correlation that can't be overlooked in this context is the one between regular physical exercise and improved sleep quality. According to a study published in the Journal of Sleep Research, people who engage in regular physical activity experience better sleep quality compared to those who live a sedentary lifestyle.

Sleep, as we know, is a vital physiological process that allows our body and mind to rest, repair, and rejuvenate. Quality sleep is essential not just for physical health but also for cognitive functioning and overall mental well-being. It helps consolidate memories, enhance concentration, stimulate creativity, and maintain mood stability, among other cognitive functions. Poor sleep, on the other hand, can lead to fatigue, impaired judgment, increased stress levels, and can even exacerbate symptoms of mental health disorders.

Incorporating regular physical activity into one's routine can help regulate sleep patterns. Exercise, particularly aerobic exercises like running, cycling, or swimming, increases the amount of slow-wave sleep—an important sleep phase for memory and learning—that a person gets.

Additionally, exercise can also help manage sleep disorders such as insomnia and sleep apnea. The increase in body temperature following a workout session, followed by a gradual decrease, can promote feelings of drowsiness, helping individuals fall asleep faster and enjoy more restful sleep. Exercise also aids in reducing anxiety and depressive symptoms, further facilitating better sleep.

Moreover, exercise can help reset the body's circadian rhythm, our internal biological clock that regulates various physiological processes, including the sleep-wake cycle. Regular physical activity, especially when done outdoors (due to the exposure to natural light), can help reinforce our natural circadian rhythms, promoting more regular sleep patterns.

However, it's worth noting that timing is essential when it comes to exercising for better sleep. It's generally advised not to engage in vigorous exercise too close to bedtime, as the endorphin rush can actually make it harder to fall asleep. Instead, scheduling workouts in the morning or early evening can provide the most sleep benefits.

Physical Activity and Stress: In today's fast-paced, high-pressure world, stress has become a common challenge. But did you know that regular physical activity can serve as an effective stress buster? According to a study published in the Journal of the American Osteopathic Association, regular exercise can substantially reduce levels of stress hormones, such as cortisol, in the body.

Cortisol is often referred to as the body's "stress hormone" as it's released in response to fear or stress by the adrenal glands as part of the fight-or-flight mechanism. While this response can be life-saving in certain situations, constant high levels of cortisol due to chronic stress can lead to a plethora of health issues, including mental health problems like anxiety and depression.

Regular physical activity can combat these effects by stimulating the production of endorphins - the body's natural mood lifters or 'feel good' hormones. Endorphins trigger positive feelings in the body, similar to that of morphine. They act as analgesics (i.e., they diminish the perception of pain) and sedatives, promoting a sense of calmness and well-being.

But the benefits of exercise in stress management extend beyond biochemical processes. Exercise can also serve as a distraction, allowing individuals to break away from the cycle of negative thoughts that feed stress, anxiety, and depression. This is particularly true for rhythmic, repetitive forms of exercise—such as walking, running, or swimming—that can induce a state of meditation or the so-called 'runner's high.'

Moreover, regular physical activity promotes better sleep, enhances self-esteem, and improves overall cognitive function, all of which can help individuals manage and cope with stress more effectively.

It's also important to note that the type of physical activity does not always need to be intense for you to reap the benefits. Even light activities like taking a leisurely walk or stretching can help reduce stress levels. The key lies in consistency—making physical activity a part of your routine.

These findings from various studies underscore the undeniable and pivotal role that physical fitness plays in supporting mental health and overall well-being. When you invest time and effort into nurturing your physical health, you're not just building a stronger, more resilient body. You're also bolstering your mind, cultivating resilience, improving cognitive functions, enhancing self-esteem, and warding off mental health disorders such as anxiety and depression.

In essence, it's not just about adding years to your life by preventing physical diseases; it's about adding life to your years by promoting mental well-being and enhancing the quality of life. As we journey towards fitness, let's remember that every squat, every mile run, and every yoga pose is not just a step towards a healthier body but a leap towards a healthier mind.

Recognizing Mental Health Challenges in Fitness

While the symbiotic relationship between physical and mental health is now clear, it's essential to understand that this journey to fitness isn't always a straightforward, uphill climb. Just like with any journey, there will be obstacles, detours, and bumps along the way. Mental health challenges can arise, even when you're in the pursuit of physical fitness. Recognizing these challenges is a crucial first step in effectively addressing them.

Identifying Stress and Burnout: Signs to Watch Out For

Pushing your body to its limits in the pursuit of fitness can sometimes lead to unexpected consequences. One of these is stress and, if left unchecked, could escalate into a state of burnout. However, stress and burnout aren't exclusively due to physical overexertion. They could also stem from a lack of balance in other aspects of your life, such as work, relationships, or personal issues.

Stress is your body's response to any kind of demand or threat. When you sense danger—whether real or imagined—your body's defences kick into high gear through a rapid, automatic process known as the "fight-or-flight" reaction. This stress response is your body's way of protecting you, but when it's constantly on, it could lead to more harm than good.

Burnout, on the other hand, is a state of emotional, physical, and mental exhaustion caused by excessive and prolonged stress. It occurs when you feel overwhelmed, emotionally drained, and unable to meet constant demands. As the stress continues, you begin to lose interest and motivation in maintaining your fitness routine.

Being able to identify signs of stress and burnout is vital to prevent further harm. Here are some signs to watch out for:

Persistent Tiredness or Exhaustion: One of the first and most noticeable signs of stress and burnout is a constant feeling of tiredness or exhaustion. It's beyond just feeling 'sleepy'; it's a chronic state of fatigue that doesn't improve significantly with rest. This fatigue can manifest itself physically, leaving you feeling weak, heavy, and unable to complete physical tasks that you once handled with ease. It can also show up mentally, with feelings of 'brain fog,' difficulty concentrating, and an overwhelming sense of apathy or disillusionment.

This persistent tiredness can significantly affect your fitness routine. You might find your performance dropping, as you struggle to keep up with your workouts. The weights you could lift easily before seem impossible to move now, or the cardio routine that used to energize you now only leaves you feeling more drained.

Neglecting Responsibilities: As the stress continues and burnout looms closer, there's a tendency to start neglecting responsibilities. This isn't a conscious decision, but rather a response to the overwhelming sense of exhaustion and a lack of motivation or energy to carry on as before.

In the context of fitness, this could mean missing workout sessions, not because of valid reasons like illness or necessary rest, but because of an inability to muster the energy or will to exercise. You might also start straying from your balanced diet, opting for quick, less healthy options or skipping meals altogether. This neglect extends beyond your fitness routine. It could affect other areas of your life too, like work responsibilities, personal projects, or social commitments.

Decreased Satisfaction and Accomplishment: As the stress builds up and burnout encroaches, there's a noticeable decrease in the satisfaction and sense of accomplishment you derive from your fitness routine. The workouts that used to be exhilarating start to feel more like a chore that you'd rather avoid. The fitness goals that once motivated and inspired you, no longer seem meaningful.

The progress you make may seem insignificant and any setbacks might be blown out of proportion. This diminishing sense of satisfaction can stem from physical exhaustion and a feeling of being overwhelmed, but it can also be a psychological response to constant, unrelenting stress. This lack of fulfilment and achievement can create a vicious cycle, leading to further demotivation and a general feeling of dissatisfaction.

Altered Sleeping Patterns: Stress and burnout can have a significant impact on your sleep. You might find yourself lying awake at night, even when you're physically exhausted. This insomnia can be due to a racing mind, constant worrying, or an inability to relax.

On the other hand, you might be sleeping more than usual, using sleep as a form of escape from stress or fatigue. This oversleeping often doesn't leave you feeling refreshed or energized; instead, you might wake up feeling groggy and lethargic, further compounding the sense of fatigue.

These altered sleeping patterns can greatly affect your physical health and mental well-being, leading to a decreased ability to concentrate, mood swings, and weakened immunity, all of which can hinder your fitness progress.

Changes in Appetite: When experiencing stress and burnout, you might notice significant shifts in your eating habits. For some people, stress can lead to overeating or emotional eating, where food becomes a comfort mechanism to deal with negative feelings. This can result in unwanted weight gain and potentially exacerbate feelings of guilt or shame.

Conversely, some people might experience a loss of appetite. The constant stress and emotional turmoil can make eating feel like a chore, or you may simply forget to eat due to being preoccupied with your concerns. This can lead to weight loss, decreased energy levels, and reduced physical strength, all of which can impede your fitness progress.

Frequent Mood Swings: Stress and burnout can also manifest as emotional instability. You might find yourself oscillating between feelings of irritability, anxiety, and depression more frequently than usual. One moment you could be feeling relatively fine, and the next, you might find yourself grappling with a wave of worry, anger, or despondency. These mood swings can be disconcerting and may impact your relationships, work, and overall quality of life.

These frequent mood changes can also spill over into your fitness routine, impacting your motivation, focus, and enjoyment of your workouts. Understanding that these mood swings are potentially a symptom of a deeper issue is crucial. It's important not to dismiss these feelings but to acknowledge them and seek help if necessary.

Difficulty Concentrating: High levels of stress and burnout can lead to a noticeable drop in concentration levels. Tasks that once felt easy may seem more challenging. You may find it difficult to stay focused during your workouts, often feeling like you're merely going through the motions without truly being present.

This decreased mental clarity can also extend to other areas of your life. Whether it's work, studies, or even social interactions, you may find it increasingly hard to keep your attention focused. This cognitive aspect of burnout can not only impact your productivity but also affect your mental health, leading to feelings of inadequacy and frustration.

Physical Symptoms: Chronic stress and burnout can have visible physical manifestations too. Frequent headaches, unexplained muscle tension, upset stomach, and other physical discomforts can be your body's way of signalling that something is off balance.

For those on a fitness journey, these symptoms can pose a significant hindrance. Persistent aches and pains might decrease your workout efficiency and potentially increase the risk of injuries.

It's crucial not to ignore these physical signals. Your body is a finely tuned machine, and these signs are its way of telling you that it's time to slow down, reassess, and perhaps seek professional advice. Remember, pushing through pain is not an act of resilience but a disregard for your well-being.

"Success is walking from failure to failure with no loss of enthusiasm."

– Winston S. Churchill

Chapter - 8

Fitness and Body Image: The Fine Line Between Health and Obsession

In an age where chiselled physiques and sculpted curves are glorified across glossy magazine covers and social media feeds, the concept of body image takes centre stage. How we perceive our bodies, how we feel others perceive us, and the constant comparison with digitally enhanced images has become an integral part of our fitness journey. Let's delve into the complex relationship between body image and fitness, an intersection that can either be a motivating force or a debilitating obsession.

Body image is more than just what you see in the mirror. It's a multidimensional concept that includes how you perceive, think, feel, and act toward your body. Your body image encompasses your innermost thoughts and feelings about your appearance, shape, and size.

Unfortunately, body image isn't always rooted in reality. The fitness ideal that's often portrayed in media might lead to a distorted body image, where you see flaws that don't exist or exaggerate minor imperfections. This can lead to an obsessive focus on 'improving' the body through extreme fitness routines and diets, sometimes at the cost of health and well-being.

Social media plays a colossal role in shaping our perceptions of the 'perfect' body. Influencers flaunting 'flawless' figures, fitness gurus showcasing rigorous routines, and brands promoting a certain body type as the epitome of fitness can create unrealistic standards.

The constant exposure to these ideals can make you feel inadequate, fostering negative body image, and even leading to harmful behaviours like excessive exercise or disordered eating. On the flip side, social media can also be a platform for body positivity, encouraging acceptance and appreciation for all body types.

Many advertisements promote a one-size-fits-all approach, emphasizing lean muscles, flat abs, or the perfect hourglass figure as the epitome of health and attractiveness. This narrow representation of fitness can breed dissatisfaction and pressure to conform to these standards, sometimes leading to unhealthy exercise and eating patterns.

However, the fitness industry is also home to positive change. Many trainers, influencers, and organizations are now focusing on a more inclusive and diverse portrayal of fitness. The emphasis is gradually shifting from appearance to functionality, well-being, and the joy of movement. This shift recognizes that fitness is individualized and that health can look different for everyone.

Healthy vs. Obsessive Focus on Body Image: Recognizing the Difference

Striving for a healthy and fit body is an admirable goal. However, the line between a healthy focus on fitness and an obsessive pursuit of an "ideal" body can often blur.

A healthy focus on body image celebrates progress, appreciates the body's capabilities, and emphasizes overall well-being. It recognizes that fitness is a journey and that each body is unique. You work towards realistic goals, and you listen to your body's needs, respecting its limits.

On the other hand, an obsessive focus on body image is often characterized by constant dissatisfaction, extreme dieting, overtraining, and the neglect of other life areas. The pursuit of the "perfect" body overshadows the joy of exercise, and the nourishment of eating, and can lead to physical and mental health issues.

Recognizing the difference between these two approaches is essential for a fulfilling and sustainable fitness journey. Being mindful of your motivation, goals, and feelings about your body can help you maintain a balanced perspective. It's about embracing fitness as a way to enhance your life, not as a never-ending battle with your body.

Strategies for Developing a Positive Body Image

Developing a positive body image is a vital part of your fitness journey. A positive perception of your body can lead to increased confidence, happiness, and overall mental well-being. Here are some strategies to foster a healthy relationship with your body:

- **Set Realistic Goals:** Aim for achievable and personalized fitness goals rather than trying to conform to unrealistic or generic ideals.

- **Focus on Functionality:** Concentrate on what your body can do rather than just how it looks. Celebrate your strength, agility, and progress.

- **Avoid Comparison:** Every person's body is unique. Avoid comparing yourself to others, especially those portrayed in media, as it can lead to dissatisfaction.

- **Seek Professional Guidance:** If needed, work with fitness professionals who emphasize overall health and well-being over appearance.

- **Practice Mindfulness:** Engage in practices that promote a deeper connection with your body, such as yoga or meditation.

- **Surround Yourself with Positivity:** Engage with communities, friends, or social media accounts that promote body diversity and acceptance.

Dealing with Body Image Pressure in Fitness Environments

Fitness environments can sometimes be hotbeds for body image pressure. From comparing ourselves to fellow gym-goers to being inundated with advertisements showcasing "ideal" bodies, it's easy to feel overwhelmed. Here's how you can manage this pressure:

Educate Yourself:

Understand that the "perfect body" is a myth. Fitness is about personal growth, strength, and health, not just appearance. The pursuit of the "perfect body" is a notion that has permeated not just fitness culture but society at large. It's fueled by media, advertisements, and sometimes even peers, leading to unrealistic expectations and undue pressure. Educating oneself about these misconceptions is the first and vital step towards a healthier approach to fitness.

Every person's body is unique, and the concept of perfection varies vastly between cultures, times, and individuals. Understanding that there is no one-size-fits-all definition of the perfect body can be liberating. Photoshopped images and strategically shot videos often portray unrealistic body standards. Knowing how media can manipulate images helps to see beyond illusions, making it easier to reject unrealistic expectations.

Choose the Right Environment:

The environment in which you pursue your fitness goals can have a significant impact on your experience, progress, and mental well-being. If your current gym or fitness community doesn't resonate with your values or causes you to feel pressured or uncomfortable, it may be time to seek an environment that better aligns with what's important to you.

Think about what matters most to you in a fitness environment. Is it a non-judgmental atmosphere? Diversity in classes and training styles? Trainers who are sensitive to individual needs? Identify what feels most comfortable and motivating for you. Take the time to explore different gyms and fitness centres in your area. Read reviews, ask for recommendations, and visit a few places if possible. Look for places that emphasize inclusivity, community, and personalized support.

Talk About It:

If you're feeling uncomfortable, have an open conversation with your trainer or fellow fitness enthusiasts about your concerns. Communication is at the heart of any successful relationship, and this is especially true in the fitness environment. It's essential to articulate your feelings and thoughts.

Build a Support System:

The journey towards health and fitness is both exciting and challenging. Surrounding yourself with friends, family, or other like-minded individuals who share or support your perspective on fitness and body image can make the path more enjoyable and fulfilling. Consider inviting a friend or family member to join you in workouts, runs, or classes. Fitness partnerships can create accountability, make exercising more fun, and foster a sense of camaraderie and shared achievement.

Consider Professional Help if Needed:

If the pressure is affecting your mental well-being, seeking professional counselling can provide personalized strategies to cope.

These approaches are not about ignoring the physical appearance but about aligning it with a balanced perspective where health, functionality, and self-acceptance are at the forefront. It's about finding joy in the journey and embracing fitness as a holistic approach to well-being.

"The journey may be slow or tough, but the destination is worth it. Keep going and never give up."

– Kapil Mehrotra

Chapter - 9

Refit at Reefit: Redefining Age and Fitness

In a world obsessed with youth and high-paced lifestyles, the concept of ageing often carries negative connotations, especially when it comes to fitness. Many believe that age is a barrier to fitness, associating youth with vitality and old age with decline. This narrative, however, is being challenged by innovative fitness initiatives like Refit at Reefit.

Refit at Reefit is not just a fitness program; it's a revolution that aims to break the stereotypes associated with ageing and fitness. It's a community connected through a WhatsApp group, yet bonded by shared goals and passions. This is where CXOs, seasoned athletes, and fitness newbies alike find their haven, a place where age is just a number.

By emphasizing tailored fitness regimens, focusing on overall wellness, and nurturing a community spirit, Refit at Reefit is redefining what it means to grow older and stay fit. This chapter will explore the philosophy behind Refit at Reefit, its transformative journey from a simple WhatsApp group to a thriving fitness community, and the ways in which it's empowering individuals across age groups.

Challenging Age Stereotypes: Starting Fitness at 38

It's never too late to start your fitness journey! The common misconception that age is a barrier to fitness has deterred many from pursuing a healthier lifestyle later in life. Who says you can't start your fitness journey at 38, or even older? The idea that 38 is "too late" to begin working out is a myth that needs to be shattered.

Starting fitness at 38 comes with its unique challenges, such as balancing work, kids, family, and daily commuting. However, with proper time management and prioritization, you can find the perfect balance. Consulting with fitness professionals and choosing routines suitable for your body can help you overcome any physical barriers. And by finding a supportive community, setting achievable goals, and tracking progress, you can stay motivated and consistent.

The benefits of taking up fitness at 38 are numerous and significant. Regular exercise can help manage weight, enhance muscle tone, and reduce the risk of chronic diseases. Moreover, it acts as a stress reliever, enhancing mental clarity and boosting mood. It also symbolizes a commitment to self-improvement, fostering a sense of accomplishment and self-esteem.

Countless individuals have embarked on their fitness journeys later in life and reaped incredible rewards. These stories stand as living proof that age is not an insurmountable obstacle, but a number that can be embraced and celebrated.

Starting your fitness journey at 38 or even later is not a constraint but an opportunity. By challenging age stereotypes and embracing a tailored approach to fitness, you can embark on a transformative journey that enhances both your physical and mental well-being. With the right mindset, determination, and support, age becomes a mark of wisdom and experience, not a limit.

Building a Fitness Community: The Birth of Reefit

During the challenging times of the global pandemic, when most were confined to their homes, fitness became a quest for many to keep themselves healthy and resilient. That's how Reefit began—a fitness community that emerged from the desire to stay fit and connect with others who shared the same vision.

While exercising and running on the roof to keep fit, sharing personal fitness videos on social media became an inspiring act that reached friends and followers alike. What started as casual sharing soon turned into something more significant. Friends began requesting daily workout routines and sessions through virtual platforms like Zoom, and the seed for a broader community was sown.

Reefit was not merely a reaction to a global crisis but a deliberate effort to promote a healthy and active lifestyle at a time when many felt isolated and disconnected. With its vision of bringing people together, regardless of their fitness level, Reefit became more than just a fitness group. It evolved into a support system, a network of motivation, camaraderie, and shared goals.

The community's strength lies in its inclusivity and encouragement. Through organized events, challenges, and support networks, Reefit provides opportunities for individuals to push their limits, reach their fitness goals, and grow both physically and mentally. The personalized touch, understanding each member's unique needs and aspirations, fosters a sense of belonging and achievement.

Reefit's growth reflects the universal longing for connection and the timeless human need for self-improvement. It represents a collective journey towards wellness, transcending age, background, and fitness level. The community's core values resonate with anyone looking to embark on a fulfilling fitness journey, making it a welcoming space for beginners and experienced athletes alike.

Joining the Reefit community means more than just pursuing a fitness regimen; it means becoming part of a movement that cherishes health, connection, and personal growth. It's a testament to the power of human connection and the incredible things we can achieve when we come together with a shared passion and purpose.

Offering Free Services: The Benefits and Challenges

The decision to offer free fitness services within the Reefit community was a step towards inclusivity and empowerment. We wanted it to represent a dedication to holistic well-being, recognizing that health is a right, not a privilege. But like all ambitious endeavours, offering free services comes with its unique blend of benefits and challenges.

Benefits:

- **Promoting a Healthier Lifestyle:** Free access to fitness resources opens doors to those who might not otherwise be able to afford them. It transcends economic barriers, enabling individuals from all walks of life to pursue a healthier and more active lifestyle.

- **Building a Sense of Community:** By bringing people together irrespective of their financial standing, the free service fosters a sense of community and togetherness. It's a space where everyone is welcome, and everyone is equal, working toward a shared vision of wellness.

- **Enhancing Reputation:** For fitness professionals involved, providing free services can be a way of giving back to the community. It's a selfless act that resonates with many and can enhance their reputation in the broader fitness industry.

Challenges:

- **Managing Costs:** Offering services without charge means absorbing the associated costs. Whether it's equipment, venue hire, or professional time, these expenses need careful consideration and sustainable planning.

- **Attracting and Retaining Participants:** While free services might attract a diverse crowd, retaining participants and ensuring they are committed to their fitness journey can be a challenge. Engaging members in a way that inspires ongoing commitment requires creative thinking and consistent effort.

- **Ensuring Sustainability:** A program that's offered for free must also be sustainable in the long term. It requires strategic planning, potential sponsorships, and continuous efforts to maintain quality without financial returns.

The challenges are real, but they are not insurmountable.

Joining the Reefit community means more than just pursuing a fitness regimen; it means becoming part of a movement that cherishes health, connection, and personal growth. It's a testament to the power of human connection and the incredible things we can achieve when we come together with a shared passion and purpose. Reefit is not just a fitness community; it's a celebration of life, resilience, and the human spirit.

In my journey towards building this fitness empire, two facets have played a pivotal role: forging connections with industry leaders and cultivating a dedicated follower base. These elements have not only shaped my career but also transformed my understanding of success in the fitness industry.

My interaction with fitness industry leaders in India opened up a world of opportunities, insights, and mentorship. The process began with attending industry events and engaging in networking activities. But it wasn't just about handing out business cards or adding connections on LinkedIn; it was about building real, meaningful relationships.

I took the time to learn about their work, showed genuine interest in their achievements, and expressed my enthusiasm for collaboration. Professionalism and reliability were my constant companions, helping me to earn their trust and credibility. We found common ground, shared resources, and I even offered my assistance whenever possible.

These relationships weren't formed overnight; they were built on shared values, respect, and mutual understanding. The bonds I forged with these industry leaders provided me with invaluable mentorship, opened doors to unique opportunities, and paved the way for successful collaborations that were both fulfilling and mutually beneficial.

Parallel to building these professional relationships, another journey was taking shape: my path to becoming a fitness influencer. It was a challenging task that demanded dedication, innovation, and authenticity.

My first step was identifying my unique niche within the fitness sphere, a place where my expertise could shine. Next came the arduous task of consistently producing content that was not only high quality but also informative, inspiring, and engaging.

I used platforms like Instagram and YouTube to reach a wider audience, but it wasn't just about numbers. It was about fostering a community, a loyal fan base that I could connect with on a personal level. Responding to comments, sharing my fitness journey, and maintaining transparency was key to building that connection.

Being an influencer wasn't about portraying a flawless image; it was about being real. I shared my triumphs as well as my setbacks, creating a dialogue that was relatable and honest. Through authenticity and consistency, I was able to establish a bond of trust with my followers, transforming them from mere spectators to active participants in my fitness journey.

These experiences, both with industry leaders and my follower base, have been more than mere steps on my career ladder; they have been learning curves, opportunities for growth, and sources of inspiration. They've taught me that success in the fitness industry, or any industry for that matter, is not about solitary pursuits but about collaboration, community, and shared passion.

The bonds I've built and the community I've fostered are not just about business; they are relationships that enrich my life, fuel my passion, and continually motivate me to strive for excellence.

The pages of this book are more than mere words; they are an invitation, a summons to challenge stereotypes, pursue wellness in all its forms, and embrace our unique journey towards fitness, connection, and self-discovery.

But this book is not just a collection of insights; it's a call to action. It invites you to step off the treadmill of conventional thinking, to delve into your urban jungle, to discover your happiness blueprint, to unleash your inner fire, and to reflect on your own perceptions of age, fitness, and wellness. It beckons you to build your own communities, to foster connections, and to ignite your passion, all while recognizing the fine line between health and obsession.

As you turn the final page, remember that the end of this book is just the beginning of your own unique journey. Let it be filled with exploration, resilience, authenticity, and joy. Let it be a path that you walk hand in hand with others, forging bonds that nourish not just your body, but your soul. Embrace your age, your body, your community, your failures, and your triumphs.